THE ICY PATH TO WELLNESS

Exploring the Benefits of Ice Baths and Cold Plunging

Loren Solis

© Copyright 2023 - All rights reserved.

The content contained within this book may not be reproduced, duplicated or transmitted without direct written permission from the author or the publisher.

Under no circumstances will any blame or legal responsibility be held against the publisher, or author, for any damages, reparation, or monetary loss due to the information contained within this book, either directly or indirectly.

Legal Notice:

This book is copyright protected. It is only for personal use. You cannot amend, distribute, sell, use, quote or paraphrase any part, or the content within this book, without the consent of the author or publisher.

Disclaimer Notice:

Please note the information contained within this document is for educational and entertainment purposes only. All effort has been executed to present accurate, up to date, reliable, complete information. No warranties of any kind are declared or implied. Readers acknowledge that the author is not engaged in the rendering of legal, financial, medical or professional advice. The content within this book has been derived from various sources. Please consult a licensed professional before attempting any techniques outlined in this book.

By reading this document, the reader agrees that under no circumstances is the author responsible for any losses, direct or indirect, that are incurred as a result of the use of the information contained within this document, including, but not limited to, errors, omissions, or inaccuracies.

TABLE OF CONTENTS

Introduction
    Overview
        Chapter 1: A Brief History
        Chapter 2: The Physiology of Cold Exposure
        Chapter 3: Immune System Boost
        Chapter 4: Enhanced Athletic Performance
        Chapter 5: Mental Health Benefits
        Chapter 6: Improved Circulation and Cardiovascular Health
        Chapter 7: Weight Loss and Metabolism
        Chapter 8: Skin and Hair Benefits
        Chapter 9: Tips for Safely Embracing the Cold
        Chapter 10: Incorporating Cold Plunges into Your Lifestyle
    Conclusion

Chapter 1: A Brief History
    1.1 Nordic Traditions
    1.2 Ancient Greece
    1.3 Eastern Traditions
    1.4 Modern Revival

Chapter 2: The Physiology of Cold Exposure
    2.1 Vasoconstriction and Thermoregulation
    2.2 Endorphin Release & Mood Enhancement
    2.3 Brown Adipose Tissue Activation
    2.4 Enhanced Immune Function
    2.5 Norepinephrine Release & PainReduction

Chapter 3: Immune System Boost
    3.1 White Blood Cell Production
    3.2 Reduction in Inflammation
    3.3 Improved Lymphatic Circulation
    3.4 Stress Reduction and Immunity
    3.5 Enhanced Antioxidant Production

Chapter 4: Enhanced Athletic Performance
    4.1 Accelerated Recovery
    4.2 Reduced Muscle Soreness
    4.3 Enhanced Endurance
    4.4 Improved Focus and Mental Resilience

    4.5 Enhanced Cardiovascular Health
    4.6 Reduced Injury Risk
Chapter 5: Mental Health Benefits
    5.1 Stress Reduction
    5.2 Anxiety Relief
    5.3 Depression Alleviation
    5.4 Mental Clarity and Focus
    5.5 Psychological Resilience
    5.6 Sleep Improvement
Chapter 6: Improved Circulation & Cardiovascular Health
    6.1 Vasodilation and Blood Flow
    6.2 Lower Blood Pressure
    6.3 Enhanced Endothelial Function
    6.4 Reduction in Heart Rate
    6.5 Lowered Risk of Heart Disease
    6.6 Improved Oxygen Delivery
Chapter 7: Weight Loss and Metabolism
    7.1 Activation of Brown Adipose Tissue (BAT)
    7.2 Enhanced Fat Burning
    7.3 Improved Insulin Sensitivity
    7.4 Calorie Expenditure
    7.5 Appetite Regulation
    7.6 Weight Management
Chapter 8: Skin and Hair Benefits
    8.1 Skin Rejuvenation
    8.2 Improved Skin Tone
    8.3 Enhanced Circulation
    8.4 Reduced Acne and Skin Conditions
    8.5 Hair Resilience
    8.6 Scalp Health
Chapter 9: Tips for Safely Embracing the Cold.
    9.1 Start Slowly
    9.2 Consult a Healthcare Professional
    9.3 Monitor Your Body
    9.4 Hydration and Nutrition
    9.5 Gradual Progression
    9.6 Warm-Up and Cool Down
    9.7 Safety
    9.8 Know the Risks
    9.9 Follow Guidelines
Chapter 10: Incorporating Cold Plunges into Your Lifestyle
    10.1 Set a Schedule

    10.2 Start Gradually
    10.3 Mix and Match
    10.4 Build a Support System
    10.5 Keep It Fun
    10.6 Track Progress
    10.7 Combine with Other Habits
    10.8 Adapt to the Seasons
    10.9 Learn from Others
    10.10 Be Patient and Persistent
Conclusion
About the Author

INTRODUCTION

The practice of submerging oneself in ice-cold water, commonly known as an ice bath or cold plunge, has been embraced by many for its remarkable health benefits. This ancient therapeutic method, once confined to athletes and adventurers, is now gaining popularity among people from all walks of life. In this mini-book, we will delve into the science and holistic advantages of embracing the cold.

OVERVIEW

Chapter 1: A Brief History

We begin by exploring the historical roots of cold water immersion. From Nordic traditions to the ancient Greeks, people have recognized the revitalizing power of cold water for centuries.

Chapter 2: The Physiology of Cold Exposure

This chapter delves into the science behind cold plunging. We discuss the body's response to cold, including vasoconstriction and the release of endorphins, which can enhance mood and reduce pain.

Chapter 3: Immune System Boost

Cold exposure has been linked to improved immune function. We explore how taking ice baths can help your body fend off illnesses and reduce inflammation.

Chapter 4: Enhanced Athletic Performance

For athletes, ice baths can be a game-changer. We examine how cold exposure accelerates recovery, reduces muscle soreness, and enhances overall athletic performance.

Chapter 5: Mental Health Benefits

Cold water immersion is not just about physical well-being; it has profound effects on mental health too. We explore how it can reduce stress, anxiety, and depression, leading to improved psychological resilience.

Chapter 6: Improved Circulation and Cardiovascular Health

Cold plunges promote better circulation and cardiovascular health. We discuss how this can lower blood pressure, reduce the risk of heart disease, and enhance overall well-being.

Chapter 7: Weight Loss and Metabolism

The metabolic advantages of cold exposure are significant. We analyze how it can aid weight loss, boost metabolism, and improve insulin sensitivity.

Chapter 8: Skin and Hair Benefits

Cold water exposure can have surprising benefits for your skin and hair. We delve into how it can lead to a healthier complexion and shinier hair.

Chapter 9: Tips for Safely Embracing the Cold

Safety is paramount when undertaking cold water immersion. We provide practical advice on how to begin and gradually build up your tolerance.

Chapter 10: Incorporating Cold Plunges into Your Lifestyle

We discuss different ways to incorporate cold plunges into your daily routine, including cold showers, ice baths, and natural bodies of cold water.

Conclusion

In this mini-book, we'll explore the many benefits of ice baths and cold plunging, from enhanced physical and mental health to improved performance and well-being. Cold exposure, once a niche practice, is now accessible to all, and its profound advantages are undeniable. Embrace the cold, and embark on a transformative journey to better health and vitality.

CHAPTER 1: A BRIEF HISTORY

Throughout the annals of human history, the practice of immersing oneself in cold water has played a significant role in various cultures and civilizations. It's a testament to the enduring belief in the revitalizing and therapeutic power of cold water. In this chapter, we will journey through time to explore the historical roots of cold water immersion.

1.1 Nordic Traditions
The concept of cold water therapy can be traced back to the frigid regions of Northern Europe. Nordic cultures, particularly those in Scandinavia, embraced the art of winter swimming and ice bathing for generations. For them, it was not just a physical activity but also a spiritual one. Immersing in icy waters was seen as a way to cleanse the body and soul, and it was often integrated into their sauna rituals.

1.2 Ancient Greece
In ancient Greece, the father of medicine, Hippocrates, recognized the potential health benefits of cold water. He prescribed cold baths for patients to relieve various ailments, a practice known as "hydrotherapy." The ancient Greeks considered cold water immersion to be a way of invigorating the body and improving overall health.

1.3 Eastern Traditions
The historical significance of cold water therapy extends beyond Europe. In Eastern cultures, such as Japan, China, and India, cold water bathing was an integral part of their traditional healing practices. In Japan, for instance, the Shinto religion involved a ritual called "Misogi," which required participants to stand beneath cold waterfalls to purify themselves spiritually and physically.

1.4 Modern Revival
While these historical practices endured for centuries, the modern world temporarily veered away from the idea of cold water immersion. However, there was a revival of interest in the mid-20th century, particularly within the sports and fitness community. Athletes, particularly swimmers and runners, began to incorporate cold water therapy into their training regimens to enhance recovery and reduce muscle soreness. This resurgence marked a return to ancient wisdom that transcended cultural boundaries.

One key figure who played a significant role in popularizing cold immersion therapy in recent years is Wim Hof. Known as "The Iceman," Wim Hof has become a prominent figure in the world of cold exposure. His extraordinary feats of endurance and resistance to extreme cold, coupled with his method "the Wim Hof method", which combines cold exposure with specific breathing techniques, have garnered worldwide attention. Wim Hof's influence has been pivotal in rekindling interest in cold water immersion as a means to unlock physical and mental benefits.

The historical roots of cold water immersion are diverse and profound, spanning various cultures and regions. From the ice-bound lakes of the North to the ancient wisdom of Greece and the rituals of the East, the practice has persisted across millennia. It speaks to a fundamental human understanding that immersing oneself in cold water can rejuvenate the body and soul. As we move forward, we'll explore how this ancient wisdom aligns with modern scientific understanding, revealing the true and remarkable benefits of cold water immersion.

CHAPTER 2: THE PHYSIOLOGY OF COLD EXPOSURE

In this chapter, we dive into the intricate science of how the human body reacts to cold exposure, shedding light on the physiological processes that underlie the benefits of immersing oneself in cold water.

2.1 Vasoconstriction and Thermoregulation
One of the immediate responses to cold water immersion is vasoconstriction. When the body perceives cold, blood vessels near the skin's surface constrict, a process aimed at conserving heat and maintaining core body temperature. This phenomenon is not just a survival mechanism; it's also central to the health benefits of cold exposure. Constricted blood vessels improve circulation and can have a positive impact on cardiovascular health.

2.2 Endorphin Release and Mood Enhancement
Cold exposure triggers the release of endorphins, our body's natural "feel-good" chemicals. This phenomenon is often referred to as a "cold-induced high." Endorphins not only alleviate pain but also enhance mood and reduce stress. The combination of the invigorating effect of cold and the subsequent release of endorphins can lead to a profound sense of well-being and mental clarity.

2.3 Brown Adipose Tissue Activation
Brown adipose tissue (BAT), often known as "brown fat," is a unique type of fat that burns calories to generate heat. Cold exposure stimulates the activation of BAT. The energy expended in this process can contribute to weight loss and an improved metabolism. This effect has sparked interest in cold exposure as a potential tool for weight management.

2.4 Enhanced Immune Function
Cold water immersion can also give your immune system a significant boost. Exposure to cold is believed to increase the production of white blood cells, which are critical components of the immune system. This enhanced immune response can help your body fend off infections and reduce inflammation.

2.5 Norepinephrine Release and Pain Reduction
Norepinephrine, a neurotransmitter and hormone, is released in response to cold exposure. This release not only improves focus and alertness but also plays a role in pain reduction. It can be

particularly beneficial for individuals suffering from chronic pain conditions.

Understanding the physiological mechanisms at play during cold exposure is essential for appreciating its wide-ranging benefits.

Vasoconstriction, the release of endorphins, the activation of brown adipose tissue, the enhanced immune function, and the release of norepinephrine collectively contribute to the transformative effects of cold immersion on the human body.

As we continue to explore the advantages of cold exposure in the following chapters, it's clear that there's more to this practice than initially meets the eye.

CHAPTER 3: IMMUNE SYSTEM BOOST

Cold exposure has a remarkable impact on the immune system, strengthening the body's natural defenses and making it more resilient to illnesses. In this chapter, we'll explore the fascinating ways in which immersing yourself in cold water can give your immune system a significant boost.

3.1 White Blood Cell Production
One of the key ways in which cold exposure enhances the immune system is by increasing the production of white blood cells, particularly neutrophils and lymphocytes. These cells are critical components of the immune system, responsible for defending the body against infections. The cold stimulates the bone marrow to release more of these infection-fighting cells into circulation.

3.2 Reduction in Inflammation
Chronic inflammation is associated with various health issues, from autoimmune diseases to heart disease. Cold exposure triggers a natural anti-inflammatory response, helping to reduce inflammation throughout the body. By alleviating chronic inflammation, cold immersion can play a role in preventing and managing inflammatory conditions.

3.3 Improved Lymphatic Circulation
The lymphatic system, a crucial part of the immune system, relies on movement to function effectively. Cold water immersion, with its invigorating effect and vasoconstriction, enhances lymphatic circulation. This means that the system responsible for carrying immune cells and removing waste from tissues operates more efficiently, contributing to overall immune system health.

3.4 Stress Reduction and Immunity
Stress has a significant impact on the immune system. High levels of stress hormones can weaken the body's ability to defend against infections. Cold exposure, with its mood-enhancing effects and release of endorphins, helps to reduce stress. As a result, it indirectly supports the immune system by creating a less stressful environment for its proper functioning.

3.5 Enhanced Antioxidant Production
Cold exposure can lead to the production of more antioxidants in the body. Antioxidants play a vital

role in neutralizing harmful free radicals that can damage cells and weaken the immune system. This increased antioxidant production contributes to overall immune system health and resilience.

The immune system is our body's primary defense against infections and diseases. Cold exposure, through its stimulation of white blood cell production, reduction in inflammation, improvement of lymphatic circulation, stress reduction, and enhanced antioxidant production, fortifies the immune system's capabilities. As we move forward, we'll continue to uncover how cold immersion can bring comprehensive benefits to your health and well-being.

CHAPTER 4: ENHANCED ATHLETIC PERFORMANCE

Cold exposure has become a secret weapon for athletes seeking to improve their performance and recovery. In this chapter, we explore the ways in which immersing oneself in cold water can be a game-changer for athletes, from reducing muscle soreness to enhancing endurance.

4.1 Accelerated Recovery
For athletes, efficient recovery is essential.

Cold exposure has been found to accelerate the recovery process. After intense workouts or competitions, immersing in cold water can reduce muscle soreness and inflammation.

This not only allows athletes to get back to training more quickly but also helps to prevent overuse injuries.

4.2 Reduced Muscle Soreness
The reduction of muscle soreness after cold exposure is a significant advantage for athletes. Cold water immersion constricts blood vessels, which can help limit the buildup of lactic acid, one of the primary causes of post-exercise muscle soreness. This means athletes can push their limits and recover faster.

4.3 Enhanced Endurance
Exposing the body to cold water can increase its tolerance to stress. Athletes who regularly engage in cold exposure often find that they can endure more extended periods of physical exertion. This is particularly beneficial for sports that demand endurance, such as long-distance running or cycling.

4.4 Improved Focus and Mental Resilience
The mental aspect of athletic performance is equally crucial. Cold exposure, with its mood-enhancing effects and the release of endorphins, can improve an athlete's focus and mental resilience. It fosters a mindset of determination and resilience, vital for achieving peak performance.

4.5 Enhanced Cardiovascular Health

Cold exposure has been linked to improved cardiovascular health. The practice of cold immersion can lead to better circulation and heart health. Athletes can benefit from improved blood flow, which means more oxygen and nutrients delivered to muscles during exercise.

4.6 Reduced Injury Risk

Cold exposure's ability to reduce muscle soreness and inflammation can also lower the risk of injury. Athletes who incorporate cold immersion into their routine are less likely to suffer from muscle strains, tears, or other exercise-related injuries.

For athletes, the advantages of cold exposure are multifaceted. From faster recovery and reduced muscle soreness to enhanced endurance, improved mental focus, cardiovascular health, and injury prevention, cold immersion is a holistic approach to boosting athletic performance. As we delve deeper into the benefits of cold exposure, it becomes clear that it has the potential to revolutionize athletic training and competition.

CHAPTER 5: MENTAL HEALTH BENEFITS

Beyond its physical advantages, cold exposure has a remarkable impact on mental health, offering a holistic approach to achieving emotional well-being. In this chapter, we delve into the ways in which immersing oneself in cold water can reduce stress, anxiety, and depression, fostering psychological resilience and clarity.

5.1 Stress Reduction
One of the most immediate effects of cold exposure is stress reduction. The shock of cold water triggers a release of endorphins, the body's natural mood-lifters. This response not only combats stress but also leaves you with a sense of euphoria. The cold immersion experience provides a mental reset, helping individuals cope with the challenges of daily life more effectively.

5.2 Anxiety Relief
Anxiety disorders affect millions of people worldwide. Cold exposure can be a powerful tool in managing anxiety. The cold-induced endorphin release and the physical shock of cold water divert your attention from anxious thoughts, offering a welcome respite from the constant mental chatter. It provides individuals with a sense of control over their mental state.

5.3 Depression Alleviation
Depression is a pervasive mental health condition, and traditional treatments often include medication and therapy. Cold exposure, however, offers a complementary approach. The release of endorphins and the enhanced circulation resulting from cold immersion can alleviate depressive symptoms, leading to a brighter mood and a more positive outlook.

5.4 Mental Clarity and Focus
The invigorating effect of cold exposure promotes mental clarity and focus. Cold water immersion is not only a physical shock but also a mental one. It forces you to be present in the moment, enhancing mindfulness. This heightened awareness can improve concentration, decision-making, and cognitive performance.

5.5 Psychological Resilience
Cold exposure teaches psychological resilience. It challenges individuals to face discomfort and

adversity head-on. Over time, this resilience can translate into better stress management, the ability to adapt to life's ups and downs, and a greater sense of mental strength.

5.6 Sleep Improvement
Many individuals struggle with sleep disorders, and insufficient sleep can exacerbate mental health issues. Cold exposure has been found to improve sleep quality. The relaxation and reduced anxiety it offers can lead to a more restful night's sleep, which, in turn, enhances mental well-being.

Cold exposure is a powerful tool for nurturing mental health. Whether through the release of endorphins, the reduction of stress and anxiety, the alleviation of depressive symptoms, the promotion of mental clarity, the development of psychological resilience, or the improvement of sleep quality, cold immersion fosters a profound sense of well-being. As we explore further, it's evident that the mental health benefits of cold exposure are an integral part of the holistic transformation it offers.

CHAPTER 6: IMPROVED CIRCULATION AND CARDIOVASCULAR HEALTH

Cold exposure offers a unique and natural method for enhancing circulation and promoting cardiovascular health. In this chapter, we will delve into the ways in which immersing oneself in cold water can lead to improved blood flow, lower blood pressure, and reduced risk of heart disease.

6.1 Vasodilation and Blood Flow
Cold exposure triggers a fascinating response known as vasodilation. When you immerse yourself in cold water, your blood vessels initially constrict to conserve heat, but then they dilate, or expand, to counteract the cold.

This sudden expansion of blood vessels results in improved circulation. Blood flows more freely, delivering oxygen and nutrients to tissues and organs.

6.2 Lower Blood Pressure
One of the key benefits of improved circulation is lower blood pressure. As blood vessels dilate during cold exposure, it reduces resistance to blood flow. This effect can lead to a significant drop in blood pressure, which is particularly beneficial for individuals with hypertension or those at risk of heart disease.

6.3 Enhanced Endothelial Function
The endothelium, the inner lining of blood vessels, plays a critical role in cardiovascular health. Cold exposure has been shown to enhance endothelial function, improving the ability of blood vessels to relax and contract as needed. This can help prevent atherosclerosis, a condition characterized by the buildup of plaque in arteries.

6.4 Reduction in Heart Rate
Cold exposure can reduce heart rate, particularly after the initial shock of immersion.

The heart becomes more efficient in pumping blood, and the reduced heart rate can alleviate the strain on the cardiovascular system. This effect is particularly advantageous for individuals with heart conditions.

6.5 Lowered Risk of Heart Disease

The combined benefits of improved circulation, lower blood pressure, enhanced endothelial function, and a reduced heart rate all contribute to a decreased risk of heart disease.

Cold exposure can help prevent conditions like atherosclerosis, hypertension, and other cardiovascular disorders.

6.6 Improved Oxygen Delivery

Enhanced circulation ensures that vital organs receive an ample supply of oxygen. This not only improves overall health but can also benefit athletic performance, as muscles receive the oxygen they need to function optimally.

Cold exposure, with its ability to stimulate vasodilation, lower blood pressure, enhance endothelial function, reduce heart rate, and lower the risk of heart disease, is a natural and holistic approach to improving cardiovascular health. As we continue our exploration of the benefits of cold immersion, it becomes clear that the advantages extend far beyond the immediate experience of cold water.

CHAPTER 7: WEIGHT LOSS AND METABOLISM

Cold exposure has garnered attention for its potential in aiding weight loss and boosting metabolism. In this chapter, we explore the mechanisms through which immersing oneself in cold water can help shed pounds and enhance metabolic function.

7.1 Activation of Brown Adipose Tissue
One of the key mechanisms behind cold exposure's role in weight loss and metabolism is the activation of brown adipose tissue (BAT).

Brown fat, in contrast to white fat, burns calories to generate heat. When exposed to cold, BAT is stimulated, leading to increased energy expenditure. This means you burn more calories, even when at rest.

7.2 Enhanced Fat Burning
Cold exposure promotes fat burning. The cold triggers the release of norepinephrine, which stimulates the breakdown of fat cells. This process, known as lipolysis, results in the release of fatty acids into the bloodstream for energy. Cold exposure can help the body rely more on fat as a fuel source, which is beneficial for weight loss.

7.3 Improved Insulin Sensitivity
Metabolism and insulin sensitivity are closely intertwined. Cold exposure has been shown to improve insulin sensitivity, making cells more responsive to insulin. This can help regulate blood sugar levels and prevent insulin resistance, a condition associated with weight gain and type 2 diabetes.

7.4 Calorie Expenditure
The increased calorie expenditure due to cold exposure is significant. While the body works to maintain its core temperature, it burns calories to generate heat. Regular cold immersion can lead to a substantial increase in energy expenditure, contributing to weight loss.

7.5 Appetite Regulation
Cold exposure can also influence appetite regulation. It has been observed that the shock of cold can suppress appetite. Additionally, the endorphin release that often follows cold immersion can lead to a better mood, reducing the likelihood of stress-induced overeating.

7.6 Weight Management

Cold exposure, through its activation of BAT, enhanced fat burning, improved insulin sensitivity, calorie expenditure, and appetite regulation, offers a comprehensive approach to weight management. Whether you're looking to shed excess pounds or maintain a healthy weight, cold immersion can be a valuable tool in achieving your goals.

The benefits of this practice extend well beyond its invigorating effect and play a multifaceted role in supporting weight loss and metabolic function.

As we continue our journey, it becomes evident that the cold has much to offer for those seeking to improve their physical health and vitality.

CHAPTER 8: SKIN AND HAIR BENEFITS

Cold exposure offers surprising advantages for the health and appearance of your skin and hair. In this chapter, we'll delve into the ways in which immersing yourself in cold water can result in a healthier complexion, improved skin tone, and shinier, more resilient hair.

8.1 Skin Rejuvenation
Cold water immersion can rejuvenate your skin. The cold temperature constricts blood vessels, reducing redness and puffiness. Additionally, it stimulates the production of collagen, a vital protein for skin elasticity, helping to maintain a youthful appearance.

8.2 Improved Skin Tone
Cold exposure can lead to improved skin tone. It helps in tightening the pores, making them appear smaller and less noticeable. This can result in a smoother and more even complexion.

8.3 Enhanced Circulation
Cold immersion enhances blood circulation, which can be beneficial for your skin since it ensures that skin cells receive an ample supply of oxygen and nutrients, promoting overall skin health.

8.4 Reduced Acne and Skin Conditions
Cold exposure can be beneficial for individuals with acne and other skin conditions. The anti-inflammatory effect of cold water can reduce redness and irritation associated with skin issues, making it a complementary approach to skincare.

8.5 Hair Resilience
Cold water can improve the resilience and shine of your hair. Cold exposure helps to close hair cuticles, making your hair smoother and shinier. It can also reduce hair breakage and split ends, leading to healthier and more manageable hair.

8.6 Scalp Health
A healthy scalp is vital for vibrant hair. Cold water exposure can promote scalp health by improving blood flow to the hair follicles. This enhanced circulation can help stimulate hair growth and prevent issues like dandruff. Cold exposure has surprising and far-reaching benefits for your skin and hair.

From skin rejuvenation and improved skin tone to the reduction of acne and the promotion of hair resilience and scalp health, cold immersion can be a valuable addition to your skincare and haircare routines. As we continue our exploration of the advantages of cold exposure, it's clear that it offers holistic benefits for both your physical and aesthetic well-being.

CHAPTER 9: TIPS FOR SAFELY EMBRACING THE COLD

While cold exposure can offer numerous health benefits, it's essential to approach it safely and gradually. In this chapter, we'll explore tips and guidelines for safely embracing the cold, ensuring that you reap the rewards while minimizing potential risks.

9.1 Start Slowly
If you're new to cold exposure, it's crucial to start slowly. Begin with shorter exposure times and less extreme temperatures. Gradually increase the duration and intensity of your cold exposure sessions as your body acclimates.

9.2 Consult a Healthcare Professional
Before incorporating cold exposure into your routine, it's wise to consult with a healthcare professional, especially if you have preexisting medical conditions. They can provide guidance on whether cold immersion is safe for you.

9.3 Monitor Your Body
Pay close attention to how your body responds to cold exposure. If you experience extreme discomfort, pain, or any adverse reactions, such as rapid breathing or shivering, it's essential to exit the cold immediately and warm up.

9.4 Hydration and Nutrition
Staying hydrated and maintaining proper nutrition is crucial when engaging in cold exposure. Proper hydration helps regulate body temperature, and a well-balanced diet provides the necessary energy to withstand the cold.

9.5 Gradual Progression
As you become more accustomed to cold exposure, you can progressively increase the duration and intensity. However, never push yourself too hard. Listen to your body and respect your limits.

9.6 Warm Up and Cool Down
Before immersing in cold water, it's beneficial to warm up your body with light exercise or a warm shower. Afterward, take time to warm up gradually. Avoid sudden temperature changes, which can be hard on the body.

9.7 Safety
When immersing yourself in cold water such as ice baths or cold plunges for the first time, having a buddy nearby is wise.

9.8 Know the Risks
Understanding the potential risks of cold exposure is crucial. These may include hypothermia, frostbite, or complications for individuals with certain medical conditions.

Being aware of these risks allows you to take appropriate precautions.

9.9 Follow Guidelines
Follow established guidelines and recommendations for safe cold exposure practices. This includes advice on how long and how often to engage in cold immersion for optimal benefits without endangering your health.

Cold exposure can be a valuable addition to your routine when approached safely. By starting slowly, consulting with a healthcare professional, monitoring your body, maintaining proper hydration and nutrition, gradually progressing, warming up and cooling down, using safety equipment, knowing the risks, and following established guidelines, you can enjoy the numerous advantages of cold immersion while minimizing potential dangers. As we continue our exploration, you'll be well-equipped to embrace the cold with confidence.

CHAPTER 10: INCORPORATING COLD PLUNGES INTO YOUR LIFESTYLE

Making cold plunges a regular part of your lifestyle requires planning and commitment. In this chapter, we'll explore practical tips on how to seamlessly integrate cold immersion into your daily routine for lasting health and well-being benefits.

10.1 Set a Schedule
Establish a consistent schedule for your cold plunges. Whether it's in the morning to kickstart your day or in the evening for relaxation, having a routine makes it easier to incorporate cold immersion into your lifestyle.

10.2 Start Gradually
If you're new to cold plunges, start gradually and increase the frequency and duration over time. This approach allows your body to adapt and reduces the shock of the cold.

10.3 Mix and Match
Cold exposure doesn't have to be the same every time. You can mix and match cold showers, ice baths, and natural bodies of cold water to keep things interesting and varied.

10.4 Build a Support System
Share your journey with others who are interested in cold exposure. Having a community or support system can provide motivation and encouragement as you incorporate this practice into your lifestyle.

10.5 Keep It Fun
Make cold exposure enjoyable. Experiment with different cold immersion techniques, play calming music during sessions, or find ways to make it a rewarding and pleasant experience.

10.6 Track Progress
Document your cold immersion experiences. Note how you feel before and after each session. Tracking your progress can be motivating and help you see the positive impact on your health and well-being over time.

10.7 Combine with Other Habits
Integrate cold exposure with other healthy habits. For example, follow your cold plunge with stretching exercises, meditation, or deep breathing to enhance the overall benefits.

10.8 Adapt to the Seasons
Consider adjusting your cold immersion routine based on the seasons. You might naturally spend more time in cold water during hot summer months and scale back in the winter.

10.9 Learn from Others
Take inspiration from experts and those who have successfully incorporated cold exposure into their lifestyles. Their experiences and tips can guide your journey.

10.10 Be Patient and Persistent
Remember that it can take time to fully adapt to cold exposure. Be patient with yourself and stay persistent. The long-term benefits are well worth the effort.

Incorporating cold plunges into your lifestyle is a holistic approach to improving your physical and mental well-being. By setting a schedule, starting gradually, mixing and matching methods, building a support system, keeping it fun, tracking progress, combining with other habits, adapting to the seasons, learning from others, and maintaining patience and persistence, you can make cold immersion a sustainable and rewarding part of your daily life. As you continue this journey, the transformative effects of cold exposure will become an integral and cherished aspect of your lifestyle.

CONCLUSION

In our journey through the world of cold exposure, we've uncovered a myriad of physical and mental health advantages that have been appreciated for centuries and are now being embraced by modern society. From the revitalizing practices of Nordic traditions and ancient Greece to the profound effects of cold exposure on the immune system, athletic performance, mental well-being, cardiovascular health, weight management, and the aesthetic benefits for skin and hair, it's clear that the cold has much to offer.

But embracing the cold is not merely a matter of stepping into icy waters. It's a holistic approach to well-being, requiring careful consideration and a commitment to gradual progression. By understanding the science behind cold exposure and the historical roots that anchor it, we gain a deeper appreciation for its transformative potential. As you embark on your journey to embrace the cold, remember that it's not just about enduring discomfort; it's about reaping the rewards. Start slowly, seek professional guidance if needed, and always listen to your body. The mental and physical resilience developed through cold exposure can be life-changing, but it's essential to be patient with yourself and prioritize safety.

Incorporating cold plunges into your daily life isn't merely a fleeting trend; it's an enduring commitment to improved health, well-being, and vitality. Whether it's by setting a schedule, building a support system, keeping it enjoyable, or integrating cold exposure with other health practices, you can make this transformative practice a lasting and cherished part of your lifestyle.

As we conclude our exploration, it's clear that the benefits of cold exposure are both ancient and modern, profound and holistic. The cold is a powerful ally in the pursuit of better health and a richer, more fulfilling life. Embrace the cold with confidence, and let it become a guiding force on your path to wellness.

ABOUT THE AUTHOR

Hello, my name is Loren Solis and I am by no means a historian or a medical professional of any kind. I am a 34-year-old Southern Californian father of 3 boys ages 14, 9 and 4.

When I was 20 years old, I was unemployed at the time and my high school buddy got me a job doing hot tub service for his father-in-law who ran one of the biggest hot tub companies in our little town of Big Bear Lake CA.

After a couple of years of that, I moved down to the South Bay Area (Redondo Beach/Torrance CA.) for a change of scenery and immediately went around to all the hot tub/spa companies I could find to try and get a job.

I was lucky enough to be hired by a small but great company right on Pacific Coast Highway in Torrance CA. "Classic Spa service" owned by the famous Mike Durand "the hot tub man".

He had been in the business for almost 40 years at the time and over now, starting out when he was only 19 years old building cedar tubs in the parking lot of that same building.

We only installed 1 cedar tub during my time there though, at that point, it was mostly regular maintenance/cleaning and repairs which were mostly warranty jobs for Hot Springs and Jacuzzi tubs that were sold out of Harbor Spas there in the South Bay. So the training I received to be able to do that work was amazing, and I learned everything I could about how all of the equipment inside a hot tub works, all the electrical components, the plumbing, and how to repair any issue.

Over time I learned enough to eventually open my own hot tub service and repair business in my hometown of Big Bear Lake CA. Which I operated for almost 10 years. For the last couple of those years, I was selling and installing my own brand of hot tub "Grizzly Tubs" made by a small private local Southern California manufacturer who I became very good friends with.

Things were going great and for a couple of years I was selling and installing hot tubs on a regular basis. Then when COVID hit for whatever reason there was a shortage of the resin used to make the acrylic sheets for the hot tub molds so all the big companies bought up all the remaining available material to secure their orders and smaller manufacturers like me were unable to get anything for a long time and production came to a standstill.

When this happened, I no longer had any regular service route customers since I was doing so well with sales and installations and I was so over cleaning spas, I had gotten rid of them all haha.

Although I wasn't able to get any more tubs, the whole control system inside which includes the heating system and the digital topside control panel with my personalized logo on it was made by a separate company which I still had access to. Sooo, I took advantage of that fact, took all my knowledge and resources and my first passion for woodworking, put it all together and built a custom one-of-a-kind wooden hot tub from scratch with all brand new equipment and materials which you can see on my business Instagram page @grizzly.tubs.

This tub is not like your traditional round wooden cedar tub either. I made mine rectangular and put a coat of marine-grade epoxy resin on the inside so the water doesn't actually come into contact with the wood. This prevents damage, increases insulation plus it feels and looks great, just like an acrylic tub but all you see is the beautiful wood grain.

My most recently built tub was a 24/7 recirculating cold plunge tub I made out of an old 132-gallon wine puncheon.

After doing some research on the top-selling cold plunge and ice baths/barrels on the market, I took all the best aspects of each and combined them to create what I believe could quite possibly be the *best* (and best looking) cold plunge tub on the market today!

Easy to use: traditionally in order to do an ice bath or cold plunge you would have to fill up a barrel or container with water and ice, which is only good for a couple of uses as the ice would melt and the temperature would rise by the time you wanted to do it again.

"The BuRR BarreL" is a fully contained unit that utilizes a water chiller with a recirculating pump, a filter, and an ozone generator that runs 24/7 pumping oxygen into the water via a tiny bubble stream to keep the water fresh and free of bacteria. This system allows the user to preset the water to a desired temperature as low as 32°F or higher. This is ideal as not everyone is ready to jump straight into 32°F water their first time doing a cold plunge. Being able to adjust the temperature allows you to start at a higher temperature and slowly work your way down over an interval of time which is a much easier and safer way to get your body used to cold immersion therapy.

The shape: I decided to use a large 132-gallon refurbished wine barrel for maximum comfort. Although cold plunging is amazing for your health, it isn't exactly a "comfortable" thing to do, so laying down in a bathtub shape plunge makes it even more uncomfortable, not to mention your lower body will naturally want to float up which is awkward while trying to submerge all the way and can take your concentration off the task at hand. By definition, the word plunge means to jump or dive quickly and energetically, using a large barrel allows you to do just that, making the whole process much easier and resulting in an all-around better experience. Not to mention they look great!

In order to build a great product, I wanted to do as much research as possible and find out not only about all the benefits of cold immersion therapy but also the history behind it and safely give tips and advice to people just getting into it. That's what this book is all about.

P.S. Thank you for taking the time to read my book. I really hope you enjoyed it and learned from it. Also, if you want to see me do my very first ever cold plunge in "The BuRR BarreL" after I built it, take a look at my Instagram @grizzly.tubs.

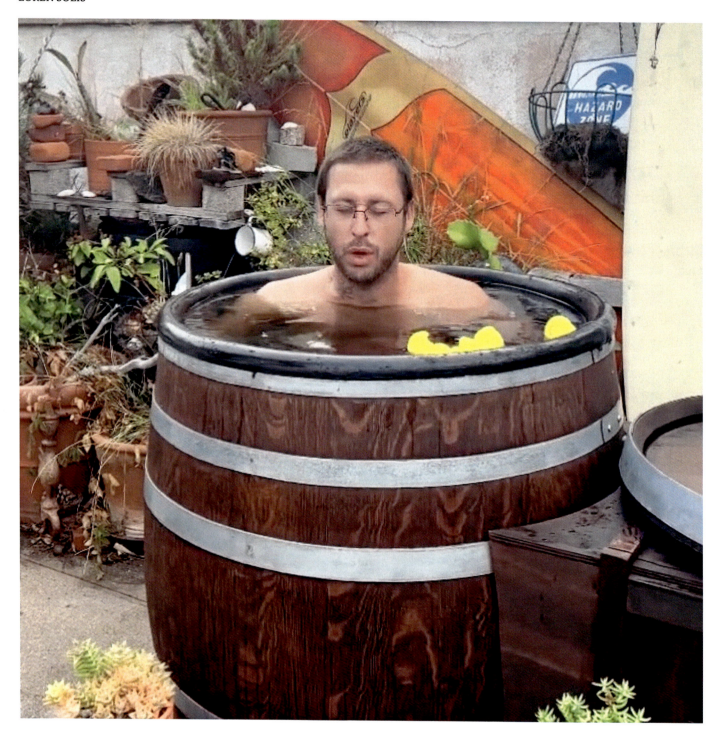

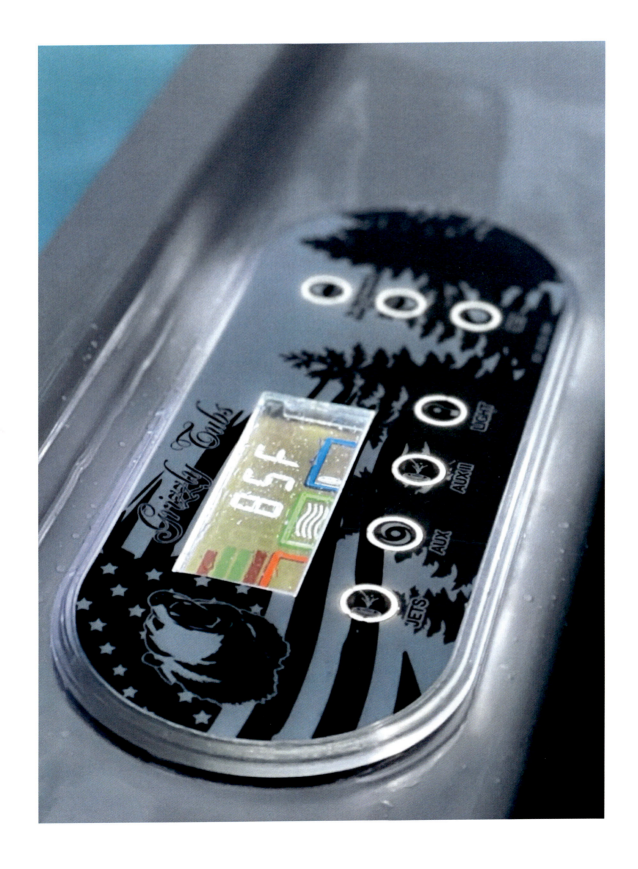

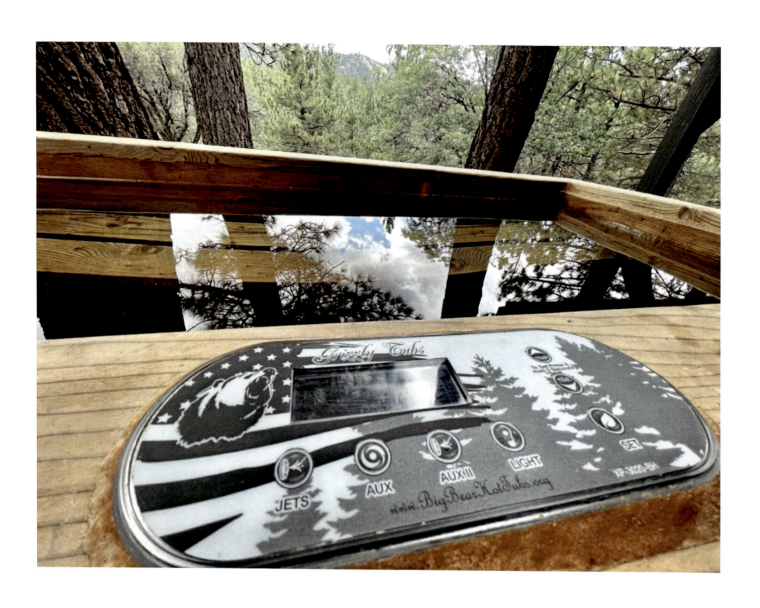

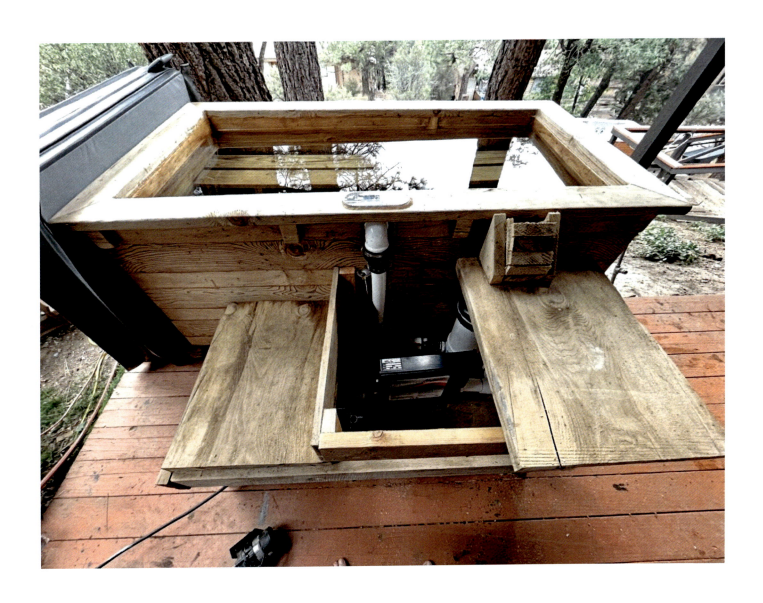

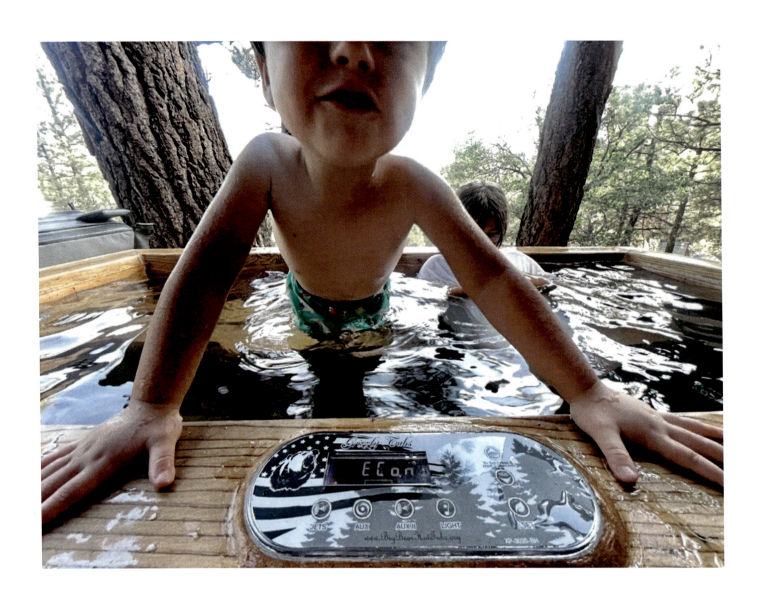

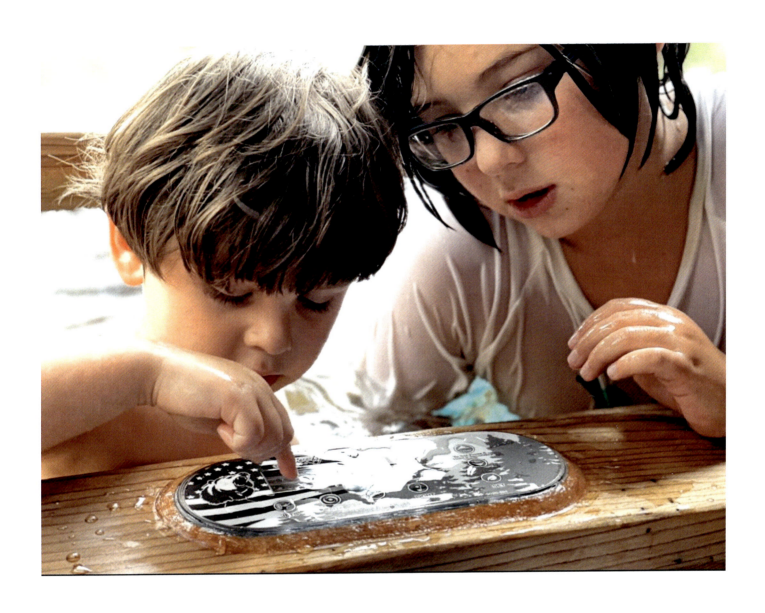

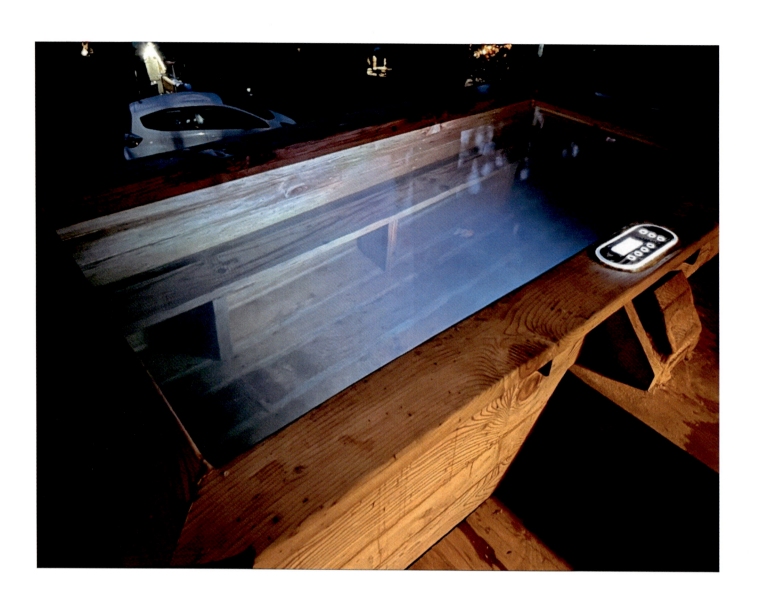

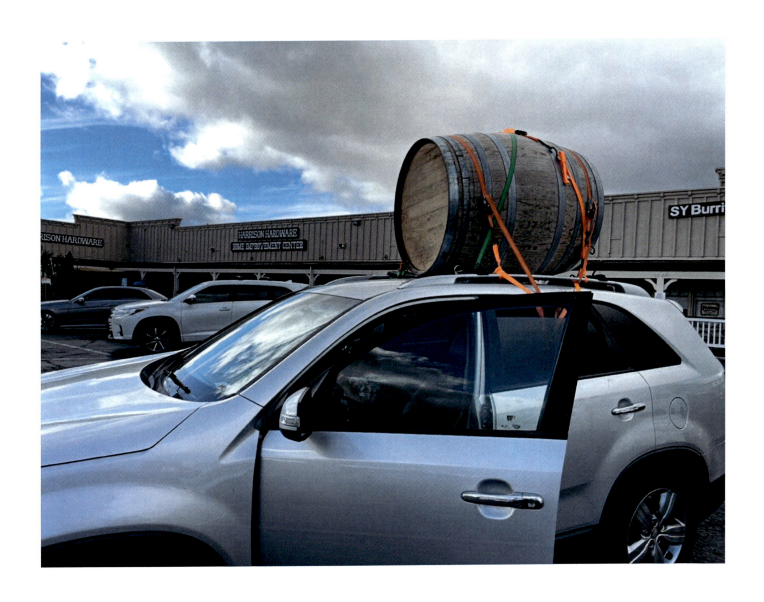

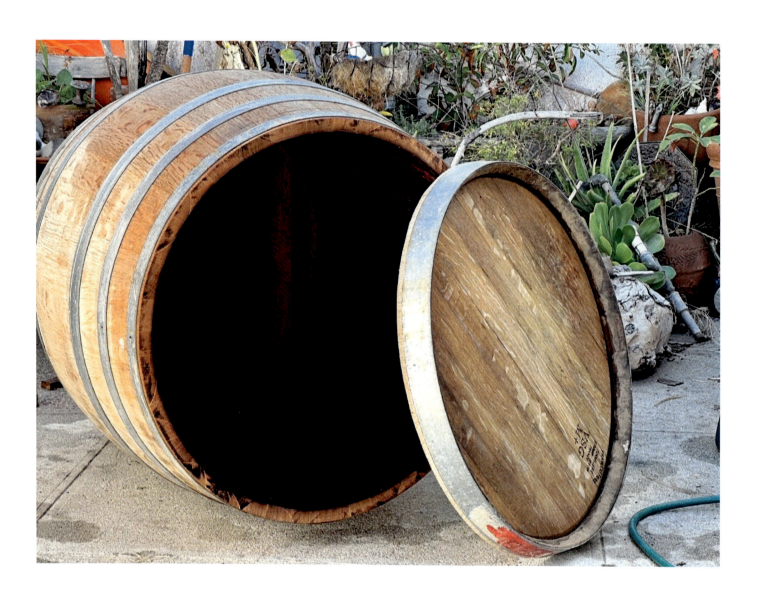

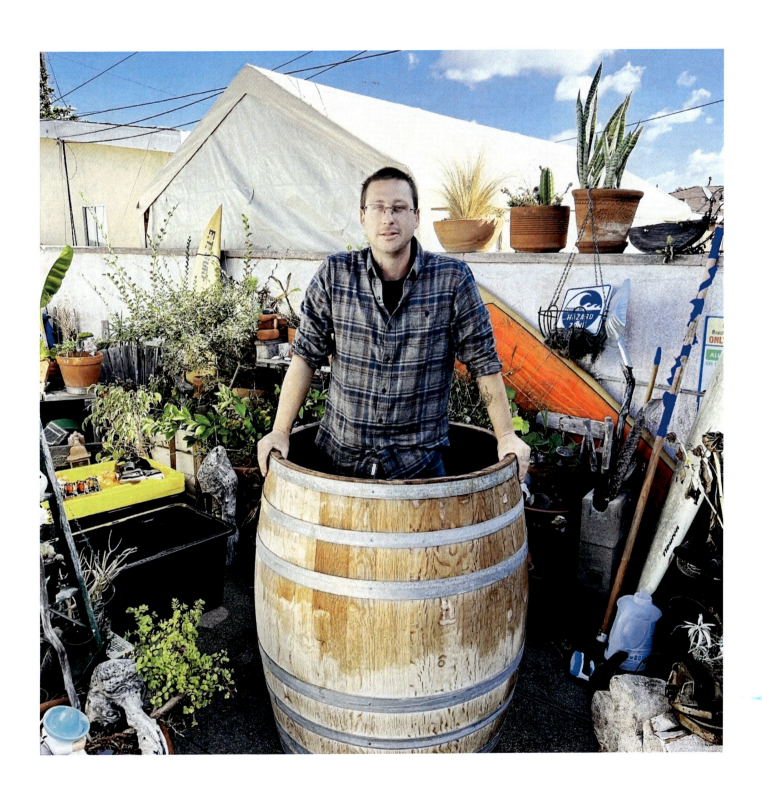

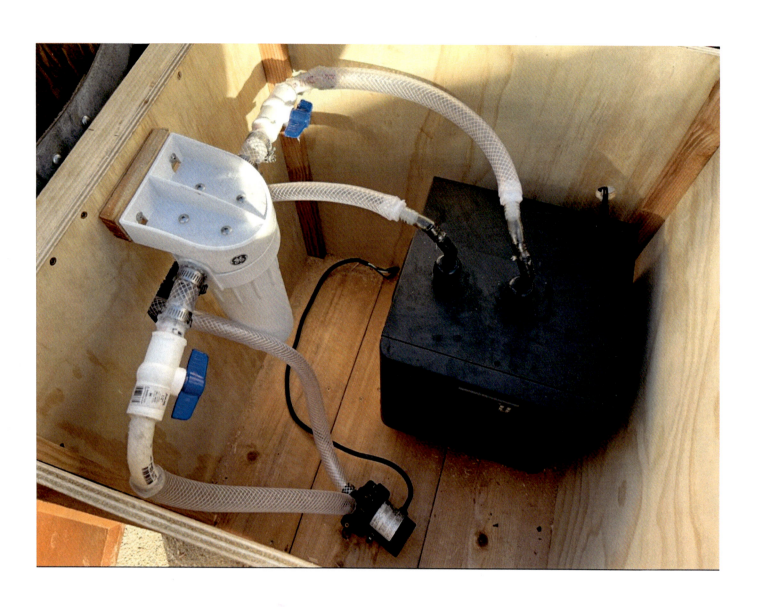

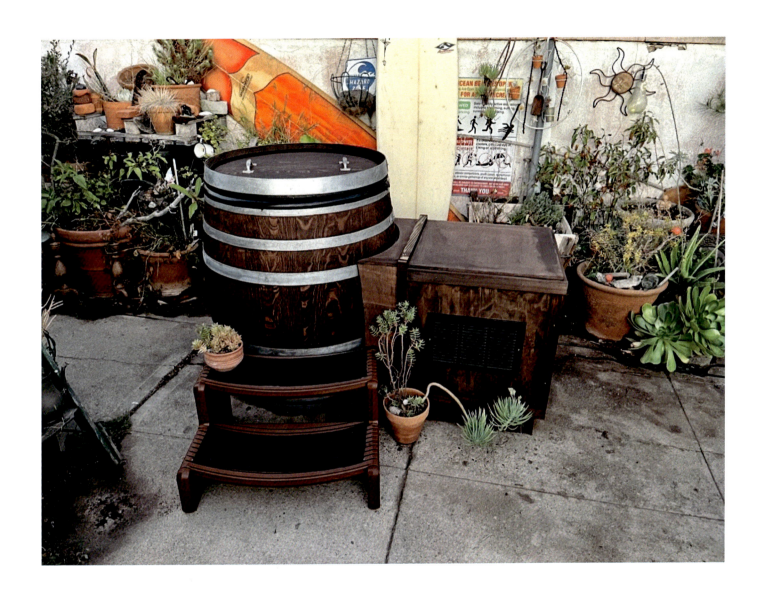

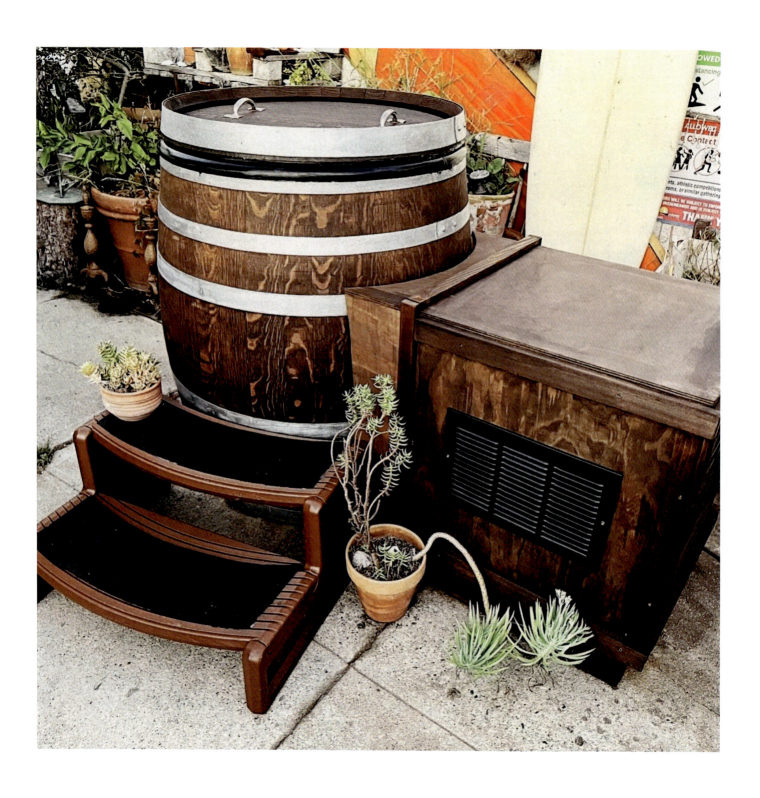

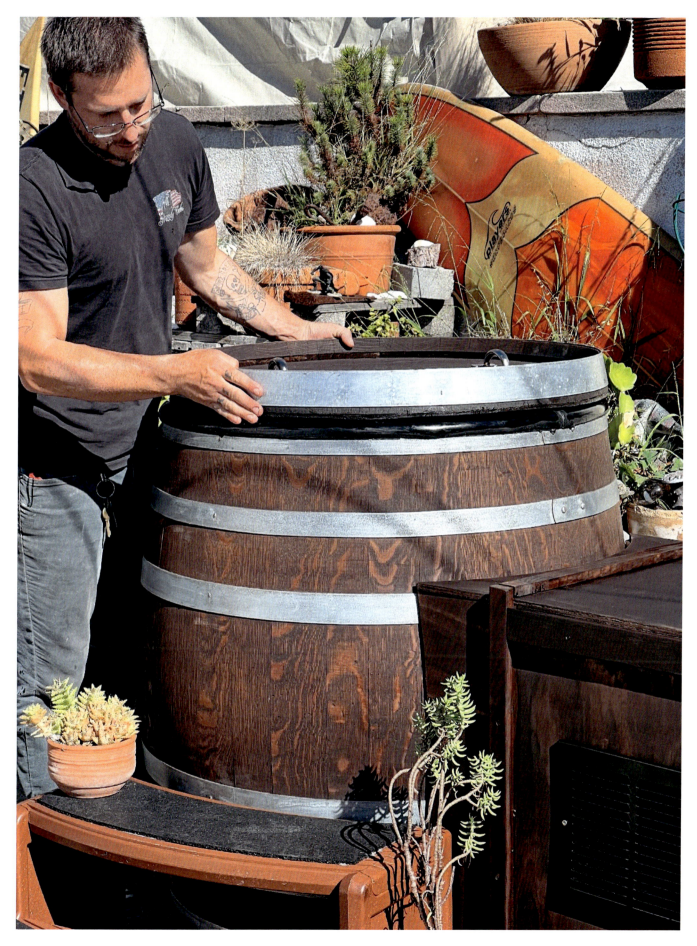

Manufactured by Amazon.ca
Acheson, AB

13544156R00029